I0434999

Health Benefits of Collard Greens

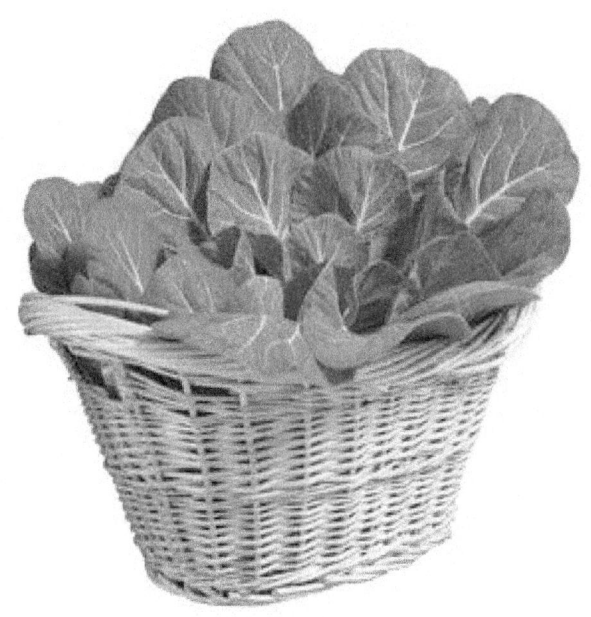

Health Benefits Series

M. Usman

Mendon Cottage Books

JD-Biz Publishing

Disclaimer

The information is this book is provided for informational purposes only. It is not intended to be used and medical advice or a substitute for proper medical treatment by a qualified health care provider. The information is believed to be accurate as presented based on research by the author.

The contents have not been evaluated by the U.S. Food and Drug Administration or any other Government or Health Organization and the contents in this book are not to be used to treat cure or prevent disease.

The author or publisher is not responsible for the use or safety of any diet, procedure or treatment mentioned in this book. The author or publisher is not responsible for errors or omissions that may exist.

Warning

The Book is for informational purposes only and before taking on any diet, treatment or medical procedure, it is recommended to consult with your primary health care provider.

Check out some of the other Healthy Gardening Series books at Amazon.com

Gardening Series on Amazon

Check out some of the other Health Learning Series books at Amazon.com

Health Learning Series on Amazon

Table of Contents

Preface

Collard greens are the green, leafy vegetables that are part of the same family as kale, broccoli and cabbage. Even though all these vegetables have the same family, they are certainly not equal in their health-promoting qualities, especially collards. See, collards have a distinct set of nutrients that enables it to step out of all the cruciferous vegetables and show its true worth. Moreover, this time tested natural drug not only does wonders for the body but is also delicious in taste.

To learn more about the vegetable, continue reading.

Getting Started

Chapter # 1: Intro

Collard greens are gaining immense respect in the nutritious-vegetables arena, mainly due to their high nutrient capacity along with low calorie density. But to understand collards, one must first understand the class of cruciferous vegetables.

Most people who even know about cruciferous vegetables associate them with vegetables like broccoli and cabbage; most of them go blank after naming these two vegetables. In recent years, research on cruciferous vegetables has skyrocketed and more people are now making them a part of their diet. Even the name cruciferous vegetables itself is undergoing an evolution. A vegetable falls under the category of cruciferous vegetables if it has four-petaled flowers that have an appearance similar to a cross or crucifix. Many scientists now prefer the name brassica vegetables over cruciferous vegetables which means "cabbage-like". The following table will ease up any difficulty you have in classifying cruciferous vegetables:

Arugula	Chinese cabbage	Horseradish
Brussels Sprouts	Cabbage	Cauliflower
Bok Choy	**Collard greens**	Radish
Broccoli	Kale	Mustard greens
Landcress	Kohlrabi	Daikon radish
Rutabaga	Turnip	Watercress

As you might know by now, collards are leafy green in appearance; they are very similar in appearance to cabbage, the only difference being the leaves of collards being loosely bound. Collards are the non-head forming member of the party and feature dark blue-green leaves that are broad in appearance and smooth in texture; unlike their cousin kale, their edges are not frilled.

They have an upright stalk that grows up to two feet in height. Collard greens are a staple in the United States and have an almost smoky flavor. They are moderately sensitive to salty soil and take 2 years to complete their biological cycle in frosty regions.

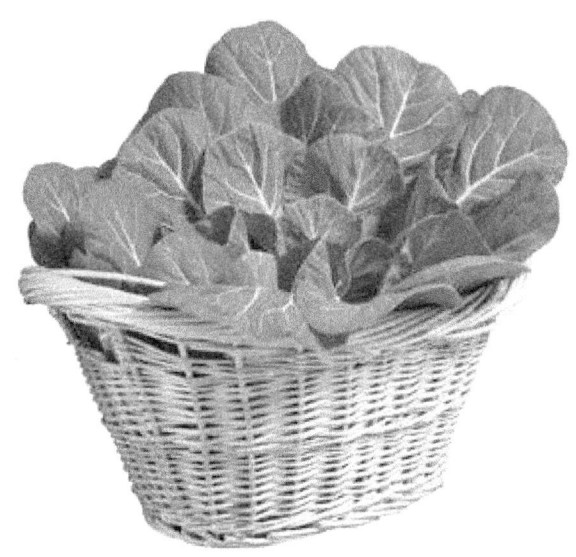

Some varieties of collard greens include:

i. **Blue Max** – These have very attractive blue-green colored leaves.

ii. **Vates** – The collard plant is compact and its leaves are smooth with dark green color.

iii. **Georgia** – Also known as Georgia Southern or Georgia LS, it is blue-green in appearance and has savoy leaves.

iv. **Flash** – It is a uniform variant of the Vates type of collards with dark green leaves.

v. **Champion** – It is a low growing variant that features smooth, green leaves.

vi.   **Heavy-Crop** – It has large, savoy, blue-green leaves.

Collards along with broccoli, kale and cauliflower are descendants of wild cabbage which can be traced as a vital food source to prehistoric times. It originated in Asia Minor and from there spread throughout Europe, thanks to groups of Celtic Wanderers. In Europe, the first known encounter with collards comes from Greek & Roman history. In the United States, collards were introduced in the 17th century; some accounts claim collard greens to be present way before the pilgrims arrived. Either way, collards have become an integral part of the world cuisine and are now enjoyed for their taste as well as nutrition.

The health benefits of collards include:

i.   **Bone Health** – Collards are excellent at repairing, as well as, strengthening bones in the body. People faced with problems like osteoporosis can greatly benefit from this vegetable.

ii.   **Blood building** – Collards being green in color, pack a lot of chlorophyll in them which helps to improve hemoglobin levels in your body. The reason being the close resemblance of chlorophyll molecules to human hemoglobin cells; thus, making it a strong contender for curing anemia. Their benefits with respect to blood include improving blood circulation and preventing stagnation in the blood.

iii.   **Cancer** – The green vegetable is also rich in antioxidants that are molecules known to ward off chemicals that cause utter destruction in the body. Not only do free radicals destroy the body externally but also aid in development of sophisticated diseases likes cancers inside the body. High levels of antioxidants can eliminate these and help lower the risk of cancer development.

iv.   **Cholesterol** – Nutrients found in collards help bring down blood cholesterol levels.

v.   **Dementia** – People with high levels of homocysteine are always at risk of diseases like dementia (Alzheimer's, Parkinson's and other cognitive ones). Collards can counter homocysteine and cause hindrance in the development of these diseases.

vi. **Heart Disease** – The same compound that prevents Parkinson's disease also prevents ailments like heart attacks and stroke. Moreover the high vitamin content stabilizes one's heart rate.

vii. **Immune System** – Vitamin C in collards helps strengthen the immune system that is necessary for maintaining the body in its optimum state.

viii. **Skin Health** – Antioxidants along with countless other nutrients improve the elasticity, firmness and health of skin in general.

ix. **Vision** – More and more UV rays are finding their way down to earth's surface and straight onto our bodies. The eyes are extremely vulnerable to these and can be damaged severely by them. Collards can supply the body with nutrients that can lower the risk of any damage caused by UV rays.

x. **Weight Loss** – Lastly, collards can both directly and indirectly help in controlling one's weight. Collards have excellent proportions of dietary fiber and chlorophyll that can give the body a feeling of satiety and improve its metabolism respectively.

The next chapter will tell you how specific nutrients in collards target health problems & ailments followed by collards' nutrient worth and how much it fulfills the body's daily requirement.

Chapter # 2: Nutritional Worth

Collard leaves are packed with a unique, health-promoting plethora of nutrients along with very low cholesterol, i.e. 30 per 100 g. That's not it; collards pack significant amounts of both soluble and insoluble fiber making them an excellent meal for diet-practitioners. Fiber is known for its satisfying properties along with protection against constipation and colorectal cancers.

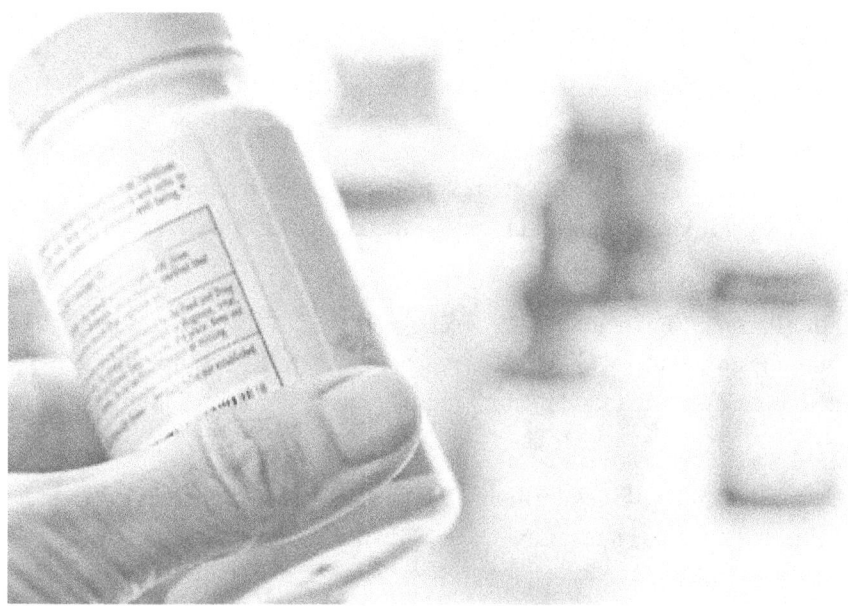

Collards are rich in invaluable supplies of phytonutrients, compounds that have lifesaving properties such as early prevention of cancer, be it prostate, colon, cervical or ovarian. There are two phytonutrients in collards that have gained immense popularity for such properties: sulforaphane and diindolylmethane with the latter having anti-bacterial, anti-viral and other immunity-boosting effects.

Collards also pack a variety of vitamins in them, namely:

- **Vitamin A** – Collards can meet up to 222% of the body's RDA per 100 grams. Vitamin A along with other carotenoids has a combined anti-oxidant effect on the body, making sure that the body remains in its top form. Some of the benefits induced by this vitamin include maintaining mucus membranes and healthy vision.

- **Vitamin C** – Vitamin C is yet another strong natural anti-oxidant that re-strengthens the body's defenses against oxidants and flu-like infections.

- **Vitamin K** – Collards pack an unbelievable amount of vitamin K in them; up to 426% of the body's daily requirement per 100 grams. Vitamin K might be the least popular vitamin out there but it plays a vital role in the body, especially at promoting osteotrophic activity and cognitive functions; it limits neuronal damage in patients of Alzheimer's disease.

- Additionally, collards are rich in B-complex vitamins like **Niacin, Pyridoxine, Riboflavin** and **Pantothenic acid**.

The leaves are also a great source of folate and that are vital for DNA synthesis and curing neural tube defects in a baby. Lastly, the leaves also contain healthy minerals like calcium, iron, manganese, copper, zinc and selenium that are each fundamental ingredients in various reactions in the body.

A detailed account of the nutritional wellness of **raw Collards** is given in the following table. The amount taken is that of a single cup or 36 grams.

Calorie Information		
Nutrient	**Amount**	**% DV**
Total Calories	10.8 (45.2 kJ)	1%
From Carbohydrates	7.4 (31.0 kJ)	
From Fat	1.3 (5.4 kJ)	
From Proteins	2.2 (9.2 kJ)	
Carbohydrates		
Nutrient	**Amount**	**% DV**
Total Carbohydrates	2.0 g	1%
Dietary Fiber	1.3 g	5%
Starch	~	

Sugar	0.2 g	

Fats & Fatty Acids

Nutrient	Amount	% DV
Total Fat	0.2 g	0%
Saturated Fat	0.0 g	0%
Mono-saturated Fat	0.0 g	
Polyunsaturated Fat	0.1 g	
Total Omega-3 Fatty acids	38.9 mg	
Total Omega-6 Fatty acids	29.5 mg	

Proteins

Nutrient	Amount	% DV
Protein	0.9 g	2%

Vitamins

Nutrient	Amount	% DV
Vitamin A	2400 IU	48%
Vitamin C	12.7 mg	21%
Vitamin E	0.8 mg	4%
Vitamin K	184 mcg	230%
Thiamin	0.0 mg	1%
Riboflavin	0.0 mg	3%
Niacin	0.3 mg	1%
Vitamin B6	0.1 mg	3%
Folate	59.8 mcg	15%
Vitamin B12	0.0 mg	0%
Pantothenic Acid	0.1 mg	1%
Choline	8.4 mg	
Betaine	0.1 mg	

Minerals

Nutrient	Amount	% DV
Calcium	52.2 mg	5%
Iron	0.1 mg	0%
Magnesium	3.2 mg	1%
Phosphorus	3.6 mg	0%

Potassium	60.8 mg	2%
Sodium	7.2 mg	0%
Zinc	0.0 mg	0%
Copper	0.0 mg	1%
Manganese	0.1 mg	5%
Selenium	0.5 mcg	1%

The following is a table stating the nutritional worth of **1 cup of collards** that have been **cooked, boiled** and then finally **drained**. The total weight of the collards is 190 grams.

Calorie Information		
Nutrient	**Amount**	**% DV**
Total Calories	49.4 (207 kJ)	2%
From Carbohydrates	33.9 (142 kJ)	
From Fat	5.7 (23.9 kJ)	
From Proteins	9.8 (41.0 kJ)	
Carbohydrates		
Nutrient	**Amount**	**% DV**
Total Carbohydrates	9.3 g	3%
Dietary Fiber	5.3 g	21%
Starch	~	
Sugar	0.8 g	
Fats & Fatty Acids		
Nutrient	**Amount**	**% DV**
Total Fat	0.7 g	1%
Saturated Fat	0.1 g	0%
Mono-saturated Fat	0.0 g	
Polyunsaturated Fat	0.3 g	
Total Omega-3 Fatty acids	177 mg	
Total Omega-6 Fatty acids	133 mg	
Proteins		

Nutrient	Amount	% DV
Protein	4.0 g	8%
Vitamins		
Nutrient	Amount	% DV
Vitamin A	15416 IU	308%
Vitamin C	34.6 mg	58%
Vitamin E	1.7 mg	8%
Vitamin K	836 mcg	1045%
Thiamin	0.1 mg	5%
Riboflavin	0.2 mg	12%
Niacin	1.1 mg	5%
Vitamin B6	0.2 mg	12%
Folate	177 mcg	44%
Vitamin B12	0.0 mg	0%
Pantothenic Acid	0.4 mg	4%
Choline	60.4 mg	
Betaine	0.2 mg	
Minerals		
Nutrient	Amount	% DV
Calcium	266 mg	27%
Iron	2.2 mg	12%
Magnesium	38.0 mg	10%
Phosphorus	57.0 mg	6%
Potassium	220 mg	6%
Sodium	30.4 mg	1%
Zinc	0.4 mg	3%
Copper	0.1 mg	4%
Manganese	0.8 mg	41%
Selenium	0.9 mcg	1%

Chapter # 3: Selection & Storage

Although collard greens are available year round in stores, they are tastier and much more nutritious in cold months, especially November through April, just after the first frost. Collards are harvested 6-8 weeks after planting and normally they are sent to the market in bunches after being cut about 4 inches from the ground. The cut ends sprout again and can be harvested again after 6-8 weeks. To ensure the best texture, some cultivators pick collards before they reach their maximum size as at this point the leaves are much thicker and less bitter in taste; it should be noted that age does not affect the flavor of the leaves.

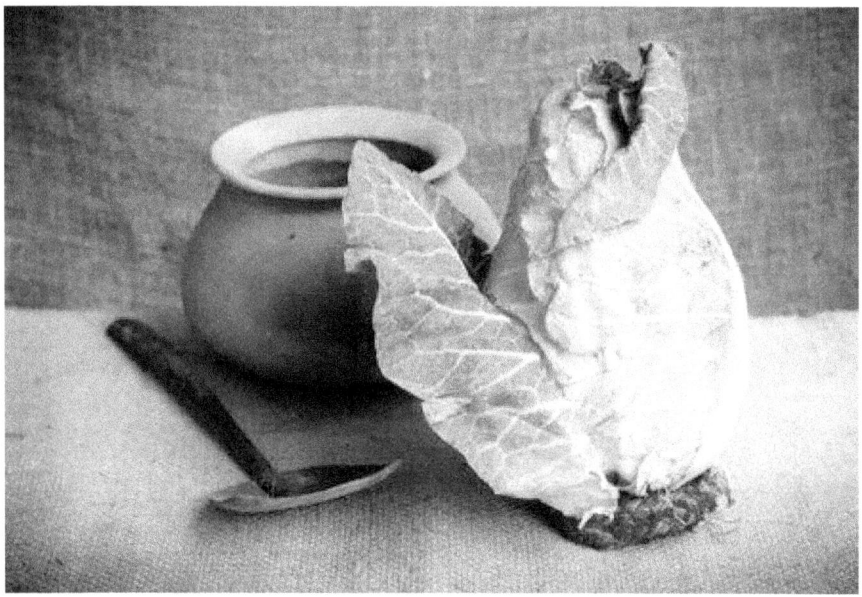

Collard greens can be enjoyed either in raw form (salads) or can be braised, sautéed, boiled or added to soups. When buying collards, choose the ones that appear to be bright, fresh and greener in color; avoid any sunken or yellow/discolored leaves as they will worsen your experience with collards. If you can, choose collards from a nearby organic farm to reap maximum benefits.

Once you get them home, wash the greens as you wash spinach. They should be washed in cold running water for sufficient time so that any dust or dirt is removed from their leaves; then rinse in salty water for about half an hour to get rid of any bacteria, germs or pesticides.

Unwashed leaves can be stored for 3 – 5 days if they are wrapped in a wet paper towel and kept in an air tight bag, however, by the passage of time, they will become bitterer and it will become a bit of a challenge to remove their tough stems. On the other hand, fresh leaves can be stored in domestic refrigerators for up to 3 days and for 10 days in high-quality freezers; the collards should still be stored in an air-tight bag. Even though collards have a much better shelf life compared to other vegetables, it is always best to consume them as soon as possible after buying as this will ensure maximum benefits going into the body.

Both the leaves and the stalk of collards are edible; the leaves must be separated from the stalk using a paring knife; the leaves can then be consumed raw or processed, but beware that extensive cooking may result in loss of nutrients like vitamin C and folate. To preserve their vitamin C content, you may cook them in a small amount of water or steam them. If you also want to preserve their original color, it's best to cook with the lid off. Also you can use the left over cooking liquid as a nutritious base for stews and soups.

Caution:

Like every other food item, collard greens must also be consumed in moderation. Despite all the health benefits they pack, eating too much of collards can cause harm to the body like swelling of the thyroid gland, etc. Furthermore, as the vegetable contains oxalic acid, it is best if sufferers of kidney stones limit their intake of the vegetable. In all cases, an average of 3 servings of collard juice should be enjoyed per week.

Health Benefits

Chapter # 1: Lowers Risk of Cancer

Cancer is probably the most well-known ailment in the modern world; it must be known that cancer is not just a single disease but rather a combination of many diseases. Cancer is the abnormal division of cells in any organ of the body. This division eventually invades other healthy tissues and contaminates the whole body. There are over 100 different types of cancer with most of them being named after the organ in which they originate respectively.

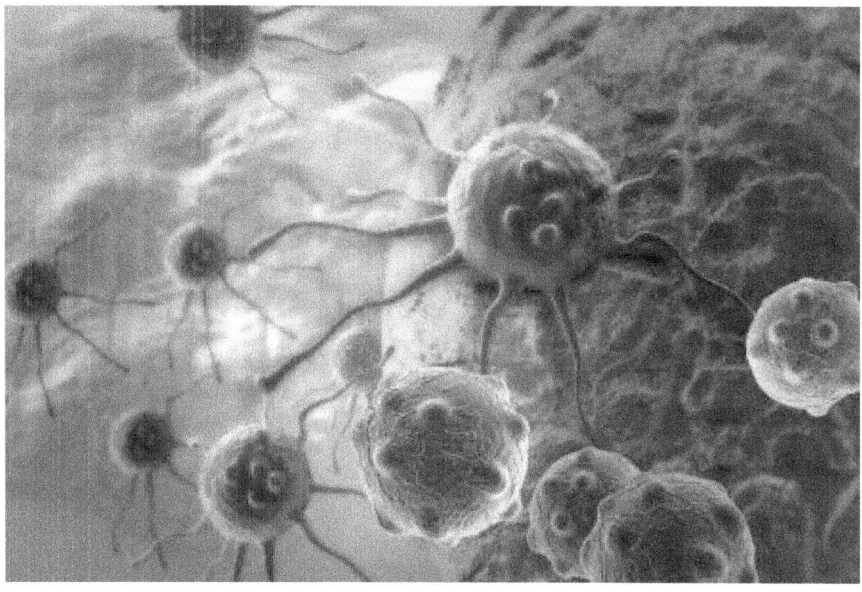

Since the 80s, special emphasis has been laid on the consumption of cruciferous vegetables, like collard greens, in order to curb a cancer outbreak. Previously it was thought that these vegetables could only lower the risk of lung and colorectal cancer, but recent studies have linked their consumption with prostate cancer as well. Furthermore, discovery of sulfur-containing compounds called *glucosinolates* in cruciferous veggies have allowed researchers to conclude that the vegetables are effective against esophageal, skin and pancreatic cancer as well. Sulforaphane, a compound formed from glucosinolates is now the area of main focus as it has been found that this particular compound proves to be most beneficial for the body in reducing the risk of cancer. Studies have shown that the compound can interfere with the development of colorectal, breast, lung and prostate cancers at different stages. A study conducted at Oregon University has shown startling results; the study was aimed at examining sulforaphane's effect on cancerous human prostate cells. It was found that that the compound not only targeted cancerous cells but also destroyed benign cells (cells at risk of becoming abnormal) and left healthy cells alone. The researchers discovered that sulforaphane inhibited HDAC enzymes that are known to cause cancer cell development. By halting the advance of HDAC enzymes, the sulfur-compound was able to prevent the spread of cancer.

It was found by researchers that when a cruciferous vegetable is chopped, cut or chewed, enzymes are released that lead to the production of sulforaphane. It was also found that cooking can decrease this content; boiling for just 9 minutes can reduce the sulforaphane content by 18%. It is best if you chew raw cruciferous vegetables that have been in storage for a short period of time. The US National Cancer Institute recommends consumption of 5 – 9 servings of vegetables & fruit per day. No official recommendation on the consumption of cruciferous vegetables has yet been launched therefore it's best to follow the general one.

In addition to *glucosinolates* collards also pack high amounts of chlorophyll that have anti-carcinogenic effects against amines that are generated when food is grilled at high temperatures e.g. bar-b-queues. These anti-cancerous effects include but are not limited to:

- Reducing the rate of oxidation in cells.
- Promoting programmed death of cancer cells.
- Reducing the production of carcinogenic molecules.
- Promoting stable DNA & cell formation.
- Bringing down any cancer-inducing gene expression.

Researchers have repeatedly shown production of carcinogens when foods are grilled at high temperatures; one of these toxins is called aflatoxin that causes liver cancer. The body is forced to absorb these harmful compounds that lead to and increase the risk of cancer. However when these compounds are combined with chlorophyll, the complex is much harder for the body to breakdown and therefore gets passed out from the body; chlorophyll is generally known for reducing the risk of liver, colon and skin cancer.

Chapter # 2: Fights Diabetes

Diabetes can strike anyone, at any time, and as a matter of fact the number of people it is bringing down is increasingly dramatically. In the last decade, the number of diabetes cases increased by 40%; almost 26 million Americans now suffer from this disease. Diabetes is taking more lives than AIDS & breast cancer combined and this should be enough to tell you about the severity of this ailment. To understand diabetes, you must first understand insulin. As you must know, the body must convert food into sugars or glucose as a fuel for the cells. After glucose has been produced, it must be soaked up by the cells and this exactly is what insulin is there for. But, for diabetics, the last part does not work correctly. Formally, diabetes is a disease that is caused by either inadequate production of blood sugar or improper response of the body to its production. There are three types of diabetes:

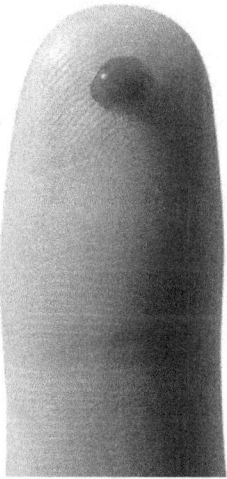

Type-1 Diabetes – The body is not able to produce insulin in adequate amounts.

Type-2 Diabetes – The body does not produce enough insulin or the cells do not respond to its production.

Gestational Diabetes – Production of insufficient glucose in pregnant women for the transport of blood sugars.

Studies have shown that type 1 diabetics who have a regular intake of high-fiber food items have lower glucose levels. In addition, type 2 diabetics can improve their blood sugar, insulin and lipid levels by inclusion of high-fiber food items, like collard greens, in their diet. As per the Dietary Guidelines for Americans, men should consume about 30-38 grams of fiber a day while women should eat about 21-25 grams of fiber a day.

Collard greens also contain an antioxidant alpha-lipoic acid that increases the body's insulin sensitivity, lowers glucose levels and prevents oxidative-stress in diabetics. Alpha-lipoic acid is in fact a natural antioxidant and is present in every cell of the body, in advance. Synthesis of this acid decreases as a person ages and is reduced further by the effect of chronic diseases. It is a necessary component in the whole energy production process due to its ability to use glucose for energy and its role in helping other antioxidants in the body. In numerous studies alpha-lipoic acid was found to be aiding in blood glucose control; it was believed that people who suffer from diabetes also suffered from peripheral neuropathy, an ailment alpha-lipoic acid can cure. In Germany, alpha-lipoic acid is even used as a prescription drug for the treatment of diabetic neuropathies. Moreover, alpha-lipoic acid can also protect against retinopathy by decreasing the risk of endothelial dysfunction in diabetics.

That's not all; the acid can also protect nerve tissues. The antioxidant is extremely useful for people who have suffered from a stroke or any dementia-related ailment. Other diseases that the antioxidant can tackle include migraines, glaucoma, multiple sclerosis, peripheral arterial disease and sun damaged skin.

Chapter # 3: Cardiovascular Support

The cardiovascular system is a collection of organs that make up for efficient transportation of nutrients inside the body and gaseous waste out of the body. It combines the heart, blood vessels, blood and a part of the lymphatic system. The cardiovascular system is quite sophisticated but at the same time quite sensitive; any damage to it can result in life threatening reactions in the body.

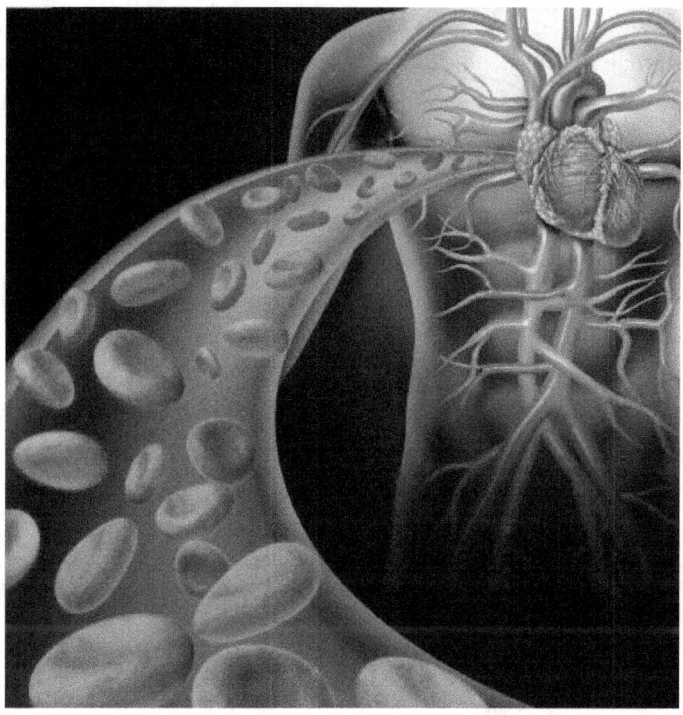

Evidence has already been found of cruciferous vegetables curing a wide array of heart problems like heart attack, atherosclerosis, heart disease and stroke. But regardless of the type of cardiovascular problem, one particular compound inside cruciferous vegetables has sparked the interest of many medical scientists, its anti-inflammatories. Previously, oxidants and other inflammatory agents were not held accountable for damages to the cardiovascular system, but new researches are showing that they do play a part in causing the anarchy and are known for creating problems, like clogging blood vessels, that leads to decreased blood flow. A specific compound in collard greens, *isothiocyanate* (ITC) sulforaphane not only triggers anti-inflammatory activity but also helps prevent as well as reverse damage to the blood vessels.

The second area where collard greens offer cardiovascular support is the cholesterol department. Cholesterol is the basic building block that is used to produce bile acids in the liver. Bile acids are molecules that aid in the absorption and digestion of fat in the body, by a process known as emulsification. These molecules are generally stored in the gall bladder along with many other acids and are released when a fat-containing meal is consumed; they are released into the intestine where they help the fat get absorbed into the body. When collards are consumed, the fiber-related nutrients bind with some bile acid molecules in the intestine so that they pass out of the body directly. This results in the liver producing new bile acid molecules and this happens by using cholesterol molecules in the body. As a result cholesterol levels go down! Collard greens can provide this benefit in both raw and cooked form. However, to reap the greatest amount of benefits, it is best to steam the collards. Collard greens are recorded to have bound as much as 46% of bile acids in the intestines in a comparison involving total dietary fiber. The collards are so good at lowering cholesterol through this mechanism that their ability is compared to a prescription drug *cholestyramine*. This should be enough to tell you the power of the mighty collard leaves.

Chapter # 4: The Little Things

Staying healthy does not mean staying protected from diseases like diabetes, cancer and heart attacks but it means living life to the fullest. While salvation from major diseases does help, really, what good is life if you suffer from sleep disorders like insomnia or cognitive impairments like memory loss? Therefore, you should not only just focus on the big problems but also make sure that the smaller ones are taken care of. That's exactly where collard greens come in.

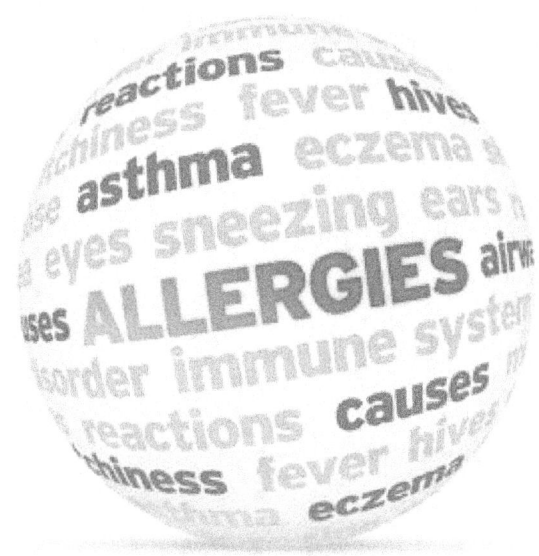

Collards are good at not only maintaining the greater part of your health but also at maintaining your muscles, cognitive approach and sleep patterns. A very beneficial nutrient inside collards known as Choline makes this all happen and helps maintain the structure of cellular membranes, transmission of nerve impulses and even the absorption of fat, among other things. Technically, choline is a vitamin-like nutrient but is mostly referred to as a

B-vitamin. Naturally, the body can produce choline in small quantities but there must be another source of choline to keep the body running smoothly.

The following are a few signs & symptoms of choline deficiency:

i.   Fatty liver

ii.   Tingling sensation in toes or fingers

iii. Fatigue

iv.   Muscle weakness

People who should be concerned the most about running low on choline include, endurance athletes, alcoholics and postmenopausal women. (The deficiency is more common in postmenopausal women than premenopausal women)

A full range of benefits of the nutrient choline found in collard greens include:

i.   Choline is necessary for the neurotransmitter responsible for the proper development of functions like:

- Memory

- Learning

- Regulation of pain

- Sleep

- Muscle movement

ii.   It controls nerve impulses and maintains the structure of cellular membranes.

iii. It is essential for the removal of not only fat but cholesterol from the body.

iv.   It acts as an anti-inflammatory and reduces chronic inflammations.

v.   Choline is a part of lung surfactant.

vi.   It plays an important role in the kidneys to balance water within the body.

vii.   It keeps patients of Alzheimer's disease safe from short-term memory losses.

viii.   It eases the symptoms of Huntington's disease.

ix.   Helps prevent gallstones.

x.   Decreases the body's sensitivity to cancerous chemicals.

Another class of very health-promoting nutrients in collards is folate. Folate is a nutrient found in many vegetables, especially collards and is vital for proper growth of the body. Sometimes known as folic acid, this nutrient helps in proper manufacturing of cells so that they have no defect. If the body gets deficient of folic acid, a condition known as megaloblastic would soon follow.

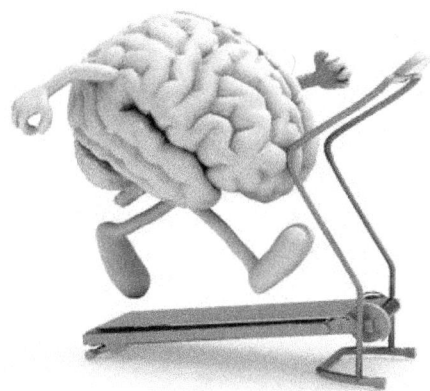

In addition, folate also helps with depression by preventing any buildup of excess homocysteine in the body, which results in a blockade of nutrients in blood from reaching many parts of the brain. Excess levels of this chemical also interferes with the positive hormones dopamine, serotonin and norepinephrine which are natural regulators of the body's mood, sleep and appetite.

All these benefits must tell you the firepower of these seemingly simple leaves; this is not the end and there are much more benefits being discovered every single day that help in raising the level of collards' popularity.

Recipes

Chapter # 1: Collard Greens with White Beans

Makes: 4 servings

Prep time: 15 minutes

Cooking time: 40 minutes

Ingredients:

- 2 tablespoons water
- 1 can unsalted diced tomatoes
- 1 ¼ cup chopped onion
- 1 ¼ cup water
- 3 tablespoons minced garlic
- Salt and ground black pepper to taste
- 1 cube beef flavored vegetarian broth
- 7 ounces collard greens
- 1 can great Northern beans, drained
- 1 teaspoon white sugar

Directions:

Place a medium skillet over medium heat and pour 2 tablespoons worth of water in it. Cook and stir the garlic and onion in the water until the onion softens and becomes translucent; add more water so as to prevent any scorching. Stir the vegetarian broth into this mixture. Then add the tomatoes, collard greens and 1 ¼ cup of water into the onion mixture and season with salt and pepper. Cover and simmer the vegetables until they become tender; this will take about 20 minutes. Stir the great Northern beans plus sugar and continue to simmer until all the liquid evaporates.

Chapter # 2: Tasty Collard Greens

Makes: 10 servings

Prep time: 30 minutes

Cooking time: 2 hours

Ingredients:

1. ¼ cup olive oil

2. 5 bunches collard greens

3. 2 tablespoons minced garlic

4. 5 cups chicken stock

5. 1 smoked turkey drumstick

6. 1 tablespoon crushed red pepper

7. Salt and black pepper

Directions:

Take a large pot and heat olive oil in it at medium heat. Add garlic and gently sauté it until it turns light brown. Add the chicken stock and turkey drumstick and cover the pot, allowing it to simmer for 30 minutes. Add the collard greens to the pot and turn up the heat to medium-high; let the greens cook for about 45 minutes, occasionally stirring them. Reduce the heat to medium and season the dish with some salt & pepper. Continue to cook until the greens become tender; this will take about 50 minutes. Drain the greens, reserving the liquid for reheating the leftovers. Add in the red pepper to taste.

Chapter # 3: Sweet & Tangy Sautéed Collard Greens

Makes: 8 servings

Prep time: 10 minutes

Cooking time: 10 minutes

Ingredients:

1. 1 tablespoon vegetable oil
2. 2 tablespoons honey
3. ½ Vidalia
4. 1 teaspoon grated ginger root
5. 1 ½ pounds collard greens
6. 5 tablespoons melted butter
7. ½ cup water
8. 3 tablespoons balsamic vinegar
9. Salt and black pepper

Directions:

Add onion to a large skillet over medium heat. Cook the onion while stirring it until it becomes soft. Add in the collard greens in small batches and stir them until they fit nicely into the skillet. Pour in the water and cook, while stirring until collards become bright green and tender; this will take about 7 minutes. Regulate heat to prevent any burning and drain.

While the collards are cooking, whisk the vinegar, butter and ginger together in a serving bowl. Add greens to a bowl and toss the dressing.

Conclusion

Collard greens have not only topped the cruciferous chart with respect to their nutritional worth, but have also set the bar very high for any vegetable trying to enter the natural-medicine market. It is a wonderful antioxidant, anti-carcinogenic and curer of diseases that are mostly overlooked by the common populace. Collards do not leave any stone unturned when it comes to boosting the body's health and they pack a toolkit that will force you to include this delicious, as well as nutritious, food into your diet.

Every single thing from definition to recipes to health benefits has been explained in detail in the book. Follow them and live a healthy life!

References

http://www.123rf.com/photo_4112456_basket-of-fresh-collard-greens.html

http://www.123rf.com/photo_13336405_fresh-collard-greens-isolated-on-white.html

http://www.123rf.com/photo_9428257_hand-holding-medicine-bottle-to-read-label.html?term=vitamins

http://www.123rf.com/photo_25866793_fresh-and-ripe-green-collard-with-clay-pot-on-brown-sack.html

http://www.123rf.com/photo_20281489_cancer-cell-made-in-3d-software.html?term=cancer

http://www.123rf.com/photo_4773306_pricked-finger.html?term=diabetes

http://www.123rf.com/photo_20688446_heart-blood-health-with-red-cells-flowing-through-three-dimensional-veins-from-the-human-circulatory.html?term=cardiovascular

http://www.fotolia.com/id/45257208

http://www.fotolia.com/id/45156048

Author Bio

Muhammad Usman is a distinguished medical graduate of Allama iqbal medical college (AIMC). He is a professional writer who has been in the field for more than 4 years. During this time he has produced 10,000+ articles, blogs and eBooks on various niches related to diseases, health, fitness, nutrition and well-being. He is a regular contributor to several journals related to medicine and surgery. He is the editor of several journals and newspapers.

Check out some of the other JD-Biz Publishing books

Gardening Series on Amazon

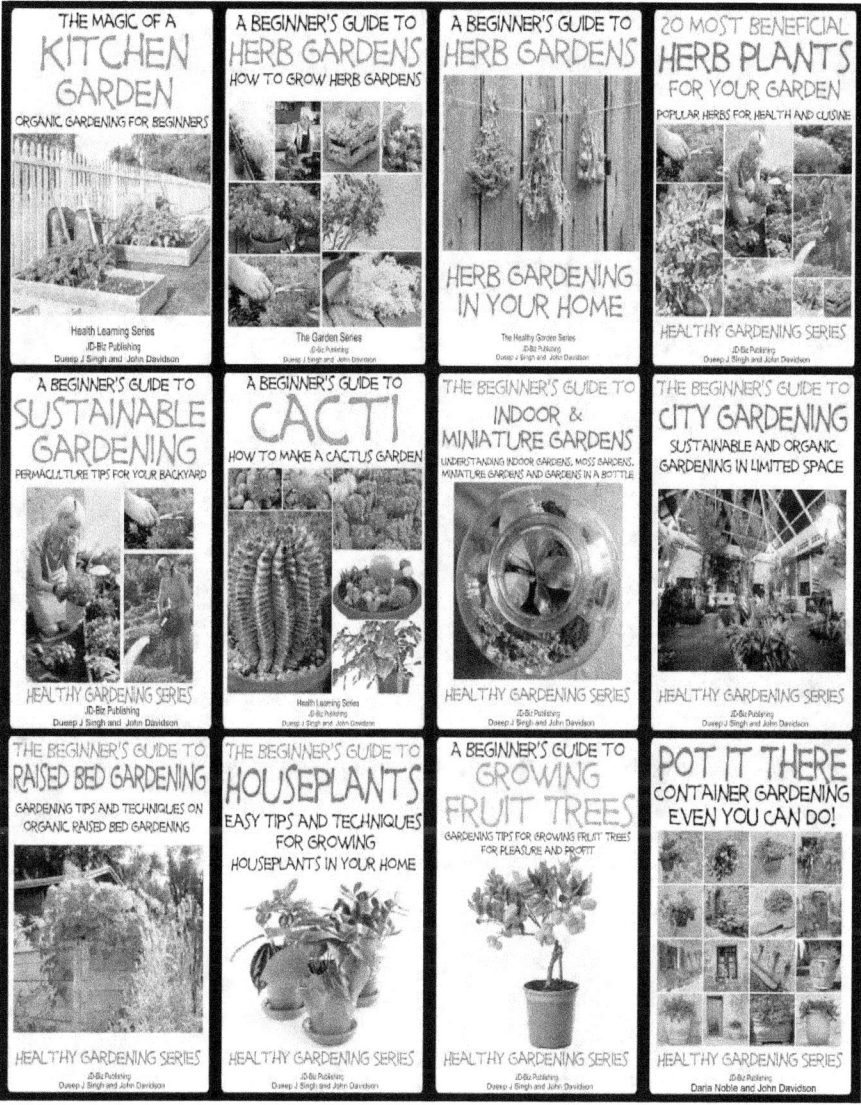

THE MAGIC OF GOOSEBERRIES FOR HEALTH AND BEAUTY
Natural Remedy Series

THE MAGIC OF YOGURT FOR COOKING AND BEAUTY
Natural Remedy Series

THE MAGIC OF LEMONS USING LEMONS FOR HEALTH AND BEAUTY
Natural Remedy Series

THE MAGIC OF CHILLIES FOR COOKING AND HEALING
Natural Remedy Series

THE MAGIC OF ONIONS ONIONS IN CUISINE TO CURE AND TO HEAL
Natural Remedy Series

THE MAGIC OF RADISHES TO CURE AND TO HEAL
Natural Remedy Series

THE MAGIC OF CARROTS TO CURE AND TO HEAL
Natural Remedy Series

THE HEALTH BENEFITS OF OREGANO FOR COOKING AND HEALTH
Natural Remedy Series

THE MAGIC OF MARIGOLDS Marigolds for Health And Beauty
Natural Remedy Series

THE HEALTH BENEFITS OF CINNAMON
Natural Remedy Series

THE MAGIC OF COCONUTS FOR COOKING & HEALTH
Health Learning Series

THE MAGIC OF CLOVES FOR HEALING AND COOKING
Health Learning Series

THE MAGIC OF ASAFETIDA FOR COOKING AND HEALING
Health Learning Series

THE MAGIC OF NEEM MARGOSA TO HEAL
Natural Remedy Series

THE MAGIC OF SALT TO HEAL AND FOR BEAUTY
Natural Remedy Series

THE MAGIC OF POMEGRANATES FOR HEALTH AND BEAUTY
Natural Remedy Series

THE MAGIC OF DRY FRUIT AND SPICES REMEDIES AND RECIPES
Natural Remedy Series

THE HEALTH BENEFITS OF TURMERIC CURCUMIN FOR COOKING AND HEALTH
Natural Remedy Series

THE MAGIC OF ALOE VERA
Natural Remedy Series

THE MAGIC OF VEGETABLES ANCIENT HEALING REMEDIES AND TIPS
Natural Remedy Series

THE HEALTH BENEFITS OF ROSEMARY FOR COOKING AND HEALTH
Natural Remedy Series

THE MAGIC OF PEPPER & PEPPERCORNS FOR COOKING & HEALING
Natural Remedy Series

THE MAGIC OF MILK, BUTTER AND CHEESE FOR COOKING & HEALING
Natural Remedy Series

THE MAGIC OF CARDAMOMS FOR COOKING AND HEALTH
Health Learning Series

THE HEALTH BENEFITS OF BLACK CUMIN FOR COOKING AND HEALTH
Natural Remedy Series

THE MAGIC OF BASIL-TULSI TO HEAL NATURALLY
Health Learning Series

THE MAGIC OF SPICES FOR HEALTH AND CUISINE
Natural Remedy Series

THE MAGIC OF ROSES FOR COOKING AND BEAUTY
Natural Remedy Series

The Miraculous Healing Powers of GINGER
Natural Remedy Series

The Miracle of HONEY
Natural Remedy Series

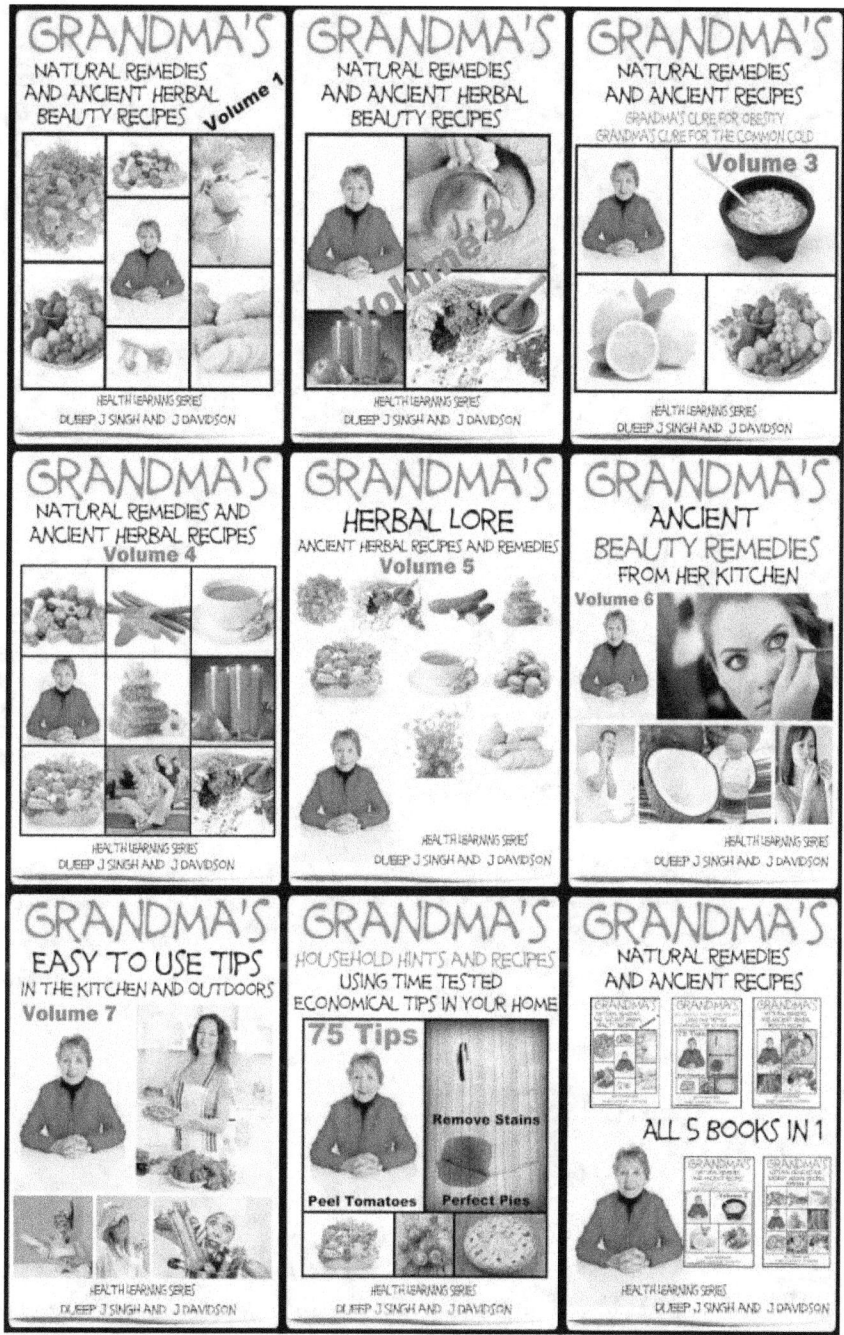

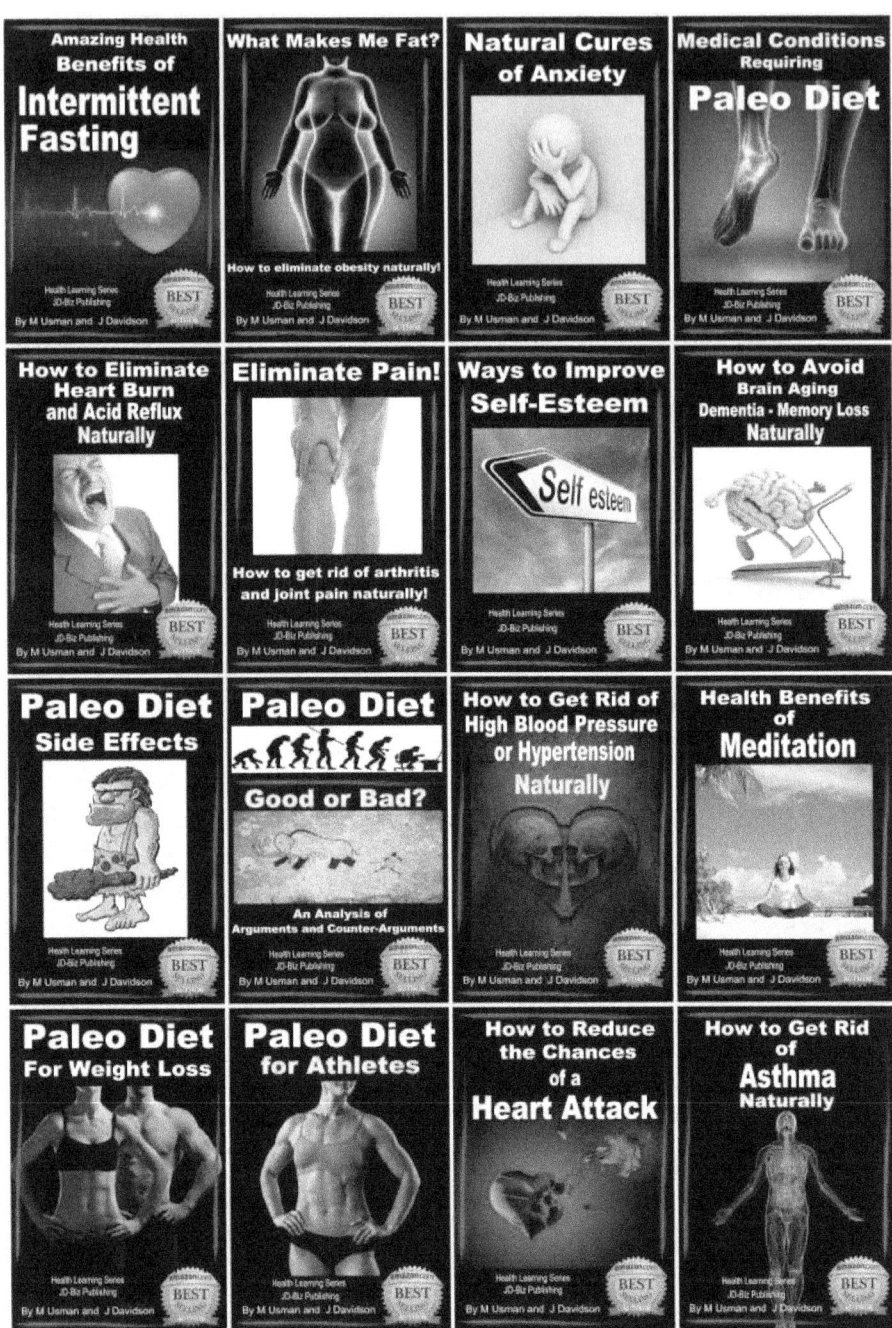

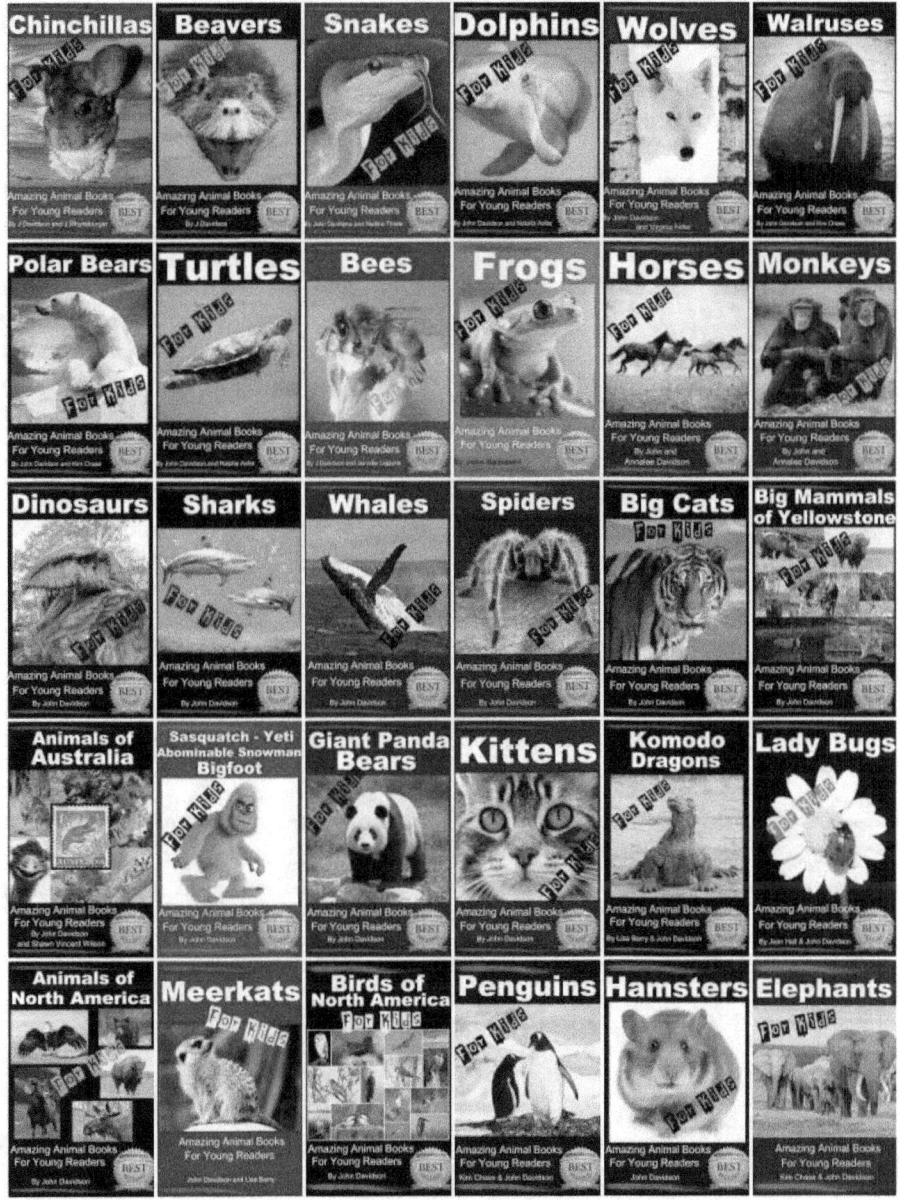

Learn To Draw Series

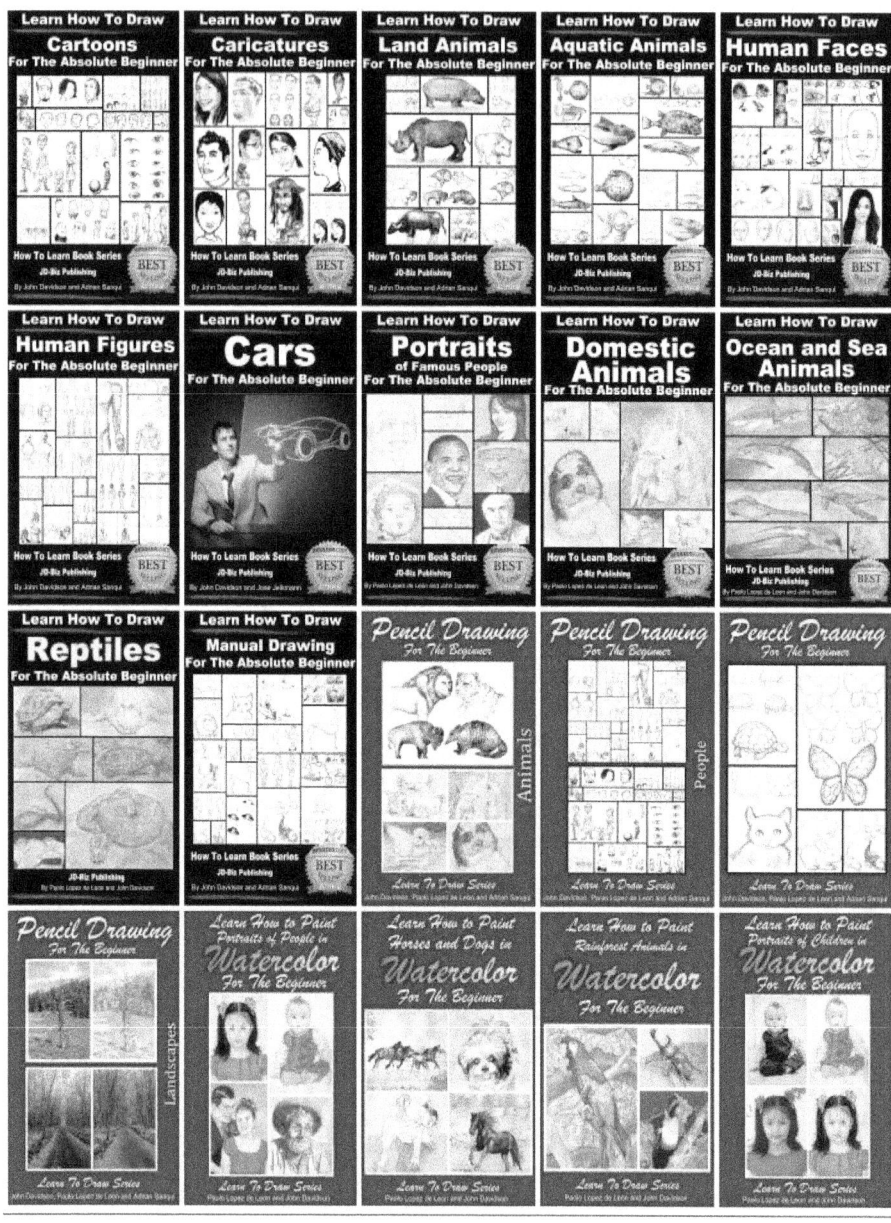

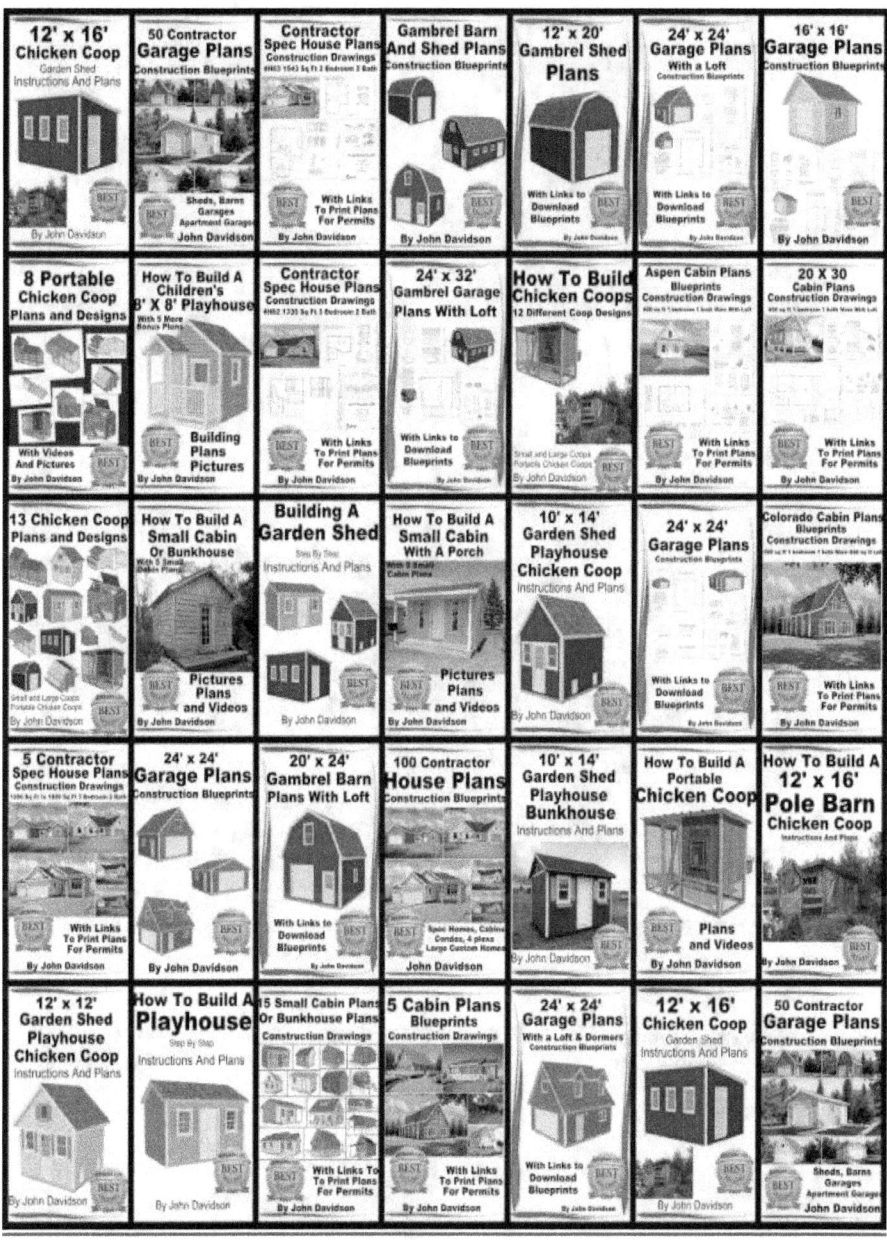

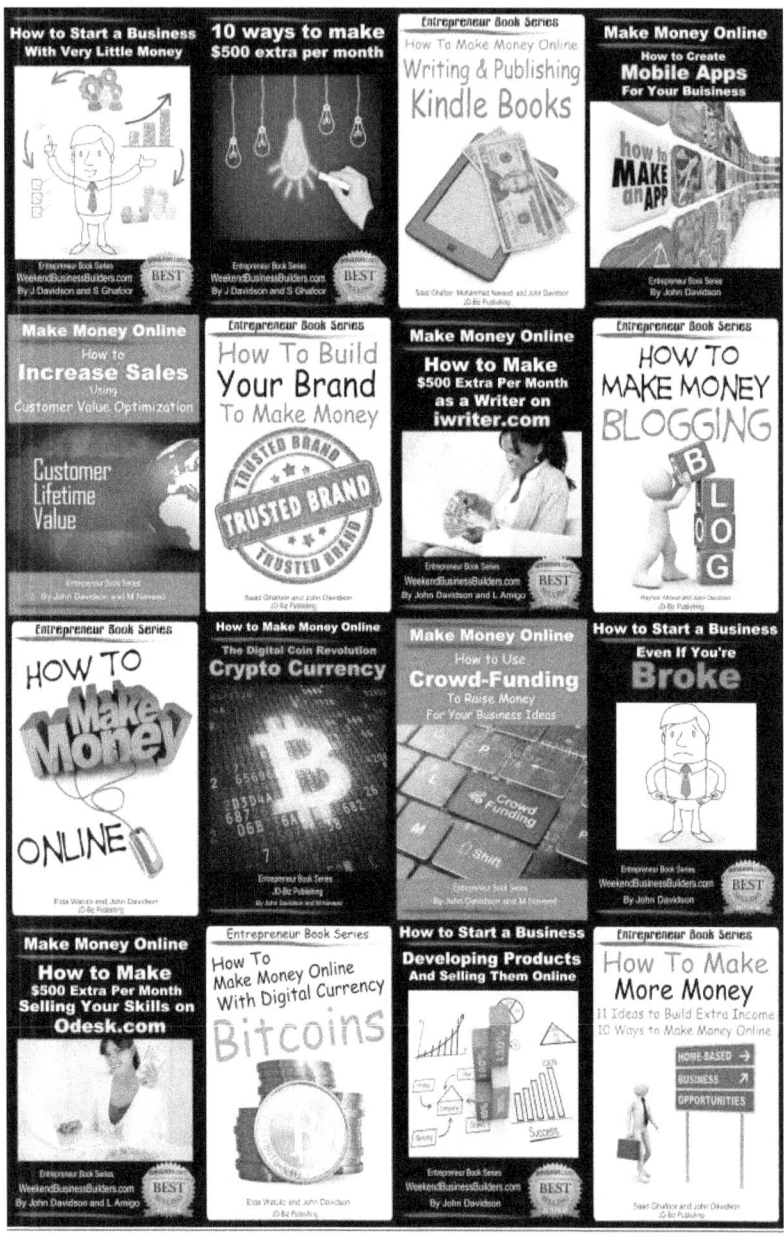

Our books are available at

1. Amazon.com

2. Barnes and Noble

3. Itunes

4. Kobo

5. Smashwords

6. Google Play Books

This book is published by

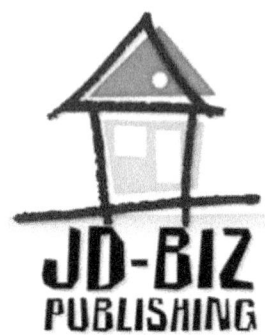

JD-Biz Corp

P O Box 374

Mendon, Utah 84325

http://www.jd-biz.com/

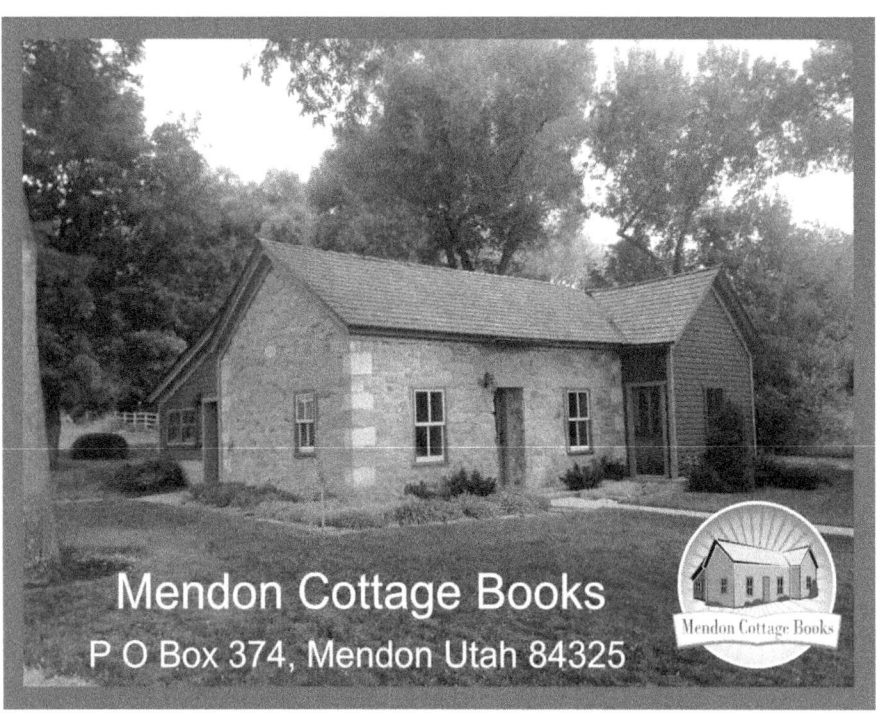

Mendon Cottage Books

P O Box 374, Mendon Utah 84325